One Month of No Sugar

Cut Down on Cravings, Restart Your Metabolism, Lose Weight, and Lower Your Blood Sugar

Koso Brown

Table of Contents

Introduction

A common feature of our contemporary lifestyle is our reliance on sugar. Sugar has gotten into everything from our typical sweets to processed snacks and sweetened beverages. However, consuming a lot of sugar has negative health impacts, such as an increased risk of heart disease, diabetes, obesity, and other chronic illnesses. Therefore, it becomes essential for our general well-being to be aware of the detrimental effects of sugar and to make deliberate decisions to limit our intake.

The amount of sugar we consume is demonstrated by the fact that data on daily sugar intake indicates that up to 65% of American adults routinely consume more sugar than is recommended by the Dietary Guidelines. Our risk of heart disease, diabetes, Alzheimer's disease, depression, and even some forms of cancer is raised by this consumption, which also leads to obesity.

Regardless of age or health situation, anyone should significantly reduce or eliminate their sugar intake; nevertheless, this does not entail eliminating all sugar. Foods containing natural sugars aren't linked to the health dangers listed above, and natural sugars can be found in fruit, some dairy products, and some vegetables. These foods also come packaged with other nutrients. When ingested in the right quantities, they are regarded as crucial elements of a healthy diet.

The sugars that are added to food during processing, manufacture, or cooking should be the ones that are focused on instead. There are various varieties of added sugars available, ranging from refined forms like corn syrup and white and brown sugar to more naturally occurring forms like honey and maple syrup. But the end effect is the same regardless of the form. When consumed in excess, added sugars can be detrimental and superfluous as they only provide calories and minimal nutrition. What occurs then if added sugars are eliminated? As it happens, the benefits extend well beyond reductions in blood sugar and weight.

Under such circumstances, is it wise to consider cutting out sugar entirely from one's diet? Furthermore, what bodily changes might someone anticipate after abstaining from sugar for a month?

This reading will explain the significance of avoiding sugar and the changes that occur in the body as a result.

Chapter 1

Consuming too much sugar

Issues arise when you eat too much added sugar, which is sugar added by food producers to their products to improve flavor or prolong their shelf life.

The majority of processed foods, soft drinks, fruit drinks, flavored yogurts, cereals, cookies, cakes, and candies are the main sources of pollution in the American diet. But foods like soups, bread, cured meats, and ketchup—which you might not consider sweetened—also contain added sugar.

We eat far too much-added sugar as a result. As per the National Cancer Institute, adult men consume 24 teaspoons of added sugar on average per day. That is equivalent to 384 cal.

"It's commonly known that eating too much sugar causes obesity and diabetes, but many men might be surprised to learn that their sweet tooth can seriously harm their heart health."

Effect on the Heart

It is unclear exactly how sugar impacts heart health, but there seem to be some indirect links. For example, excessive sugar overloads the liver. "Your liver turns food carbs into fat and metabolizes sugar in the same way as it does alcohol. This can eventually result in more fat being accumulated, which can cause fatty liver disease, which can worsen diabetes and increase your risk of heart disease. Excessive consumption of added sugar can lead to elevated blood pressure and chronic inflammation, which are pathological processes that ultimately result in heart disease. Because liquid calories are less filling than calories from solid foods, consuming too much sugar, especially in the form of sugary drinks, can also cause weight gain by deceiving your body's appetite-control mechanism. Because of this, it is simpler for people to increase the number of calories in their regular diet when they drink sugary drinks.

An increased risk of heart attack and stroke is associated with the effects of added sugar intake, including elevated blood pressure, inflammation, weight gain, diabetes, and fatty liver disease.

What Effects Does Sugar Have on Your Health?

When you ask most people about the health risks associated with sugar, they'll probably bring up weight gain and dental issues. Large sugar intakes may also increase your risk of heart disease, including coronary artery disease and stroke, as many people may not be aware.

Understanding the distinction between naturally occurring and added sugars is crucial to understanding why eating sugar can be detrimental to your heart.

Natural sugars are not associated with heart disease and can be found in whole fruits and vegetables. As the name suggests, added sugars are made when food is processed or added to food.

Table sugar, candies, and sodas are obvious examples of meals with added sugars, but you might be surprised by other foods like packaged salad dressings and pasta sauces, cereal, and yogurt that are high in added sugars. In actuality, the average American consumes more than 17 teaspoons of added sugar each day, according to the American Heart Association (AHA).

Five ways that additional sugars impair heart health

1.   **Inflammation:** Excessive added sugar intake may cause long-term inflammation of the heart and blood vessels. Both blood pressure and the risk of heart disease may rise as a result.

2.   **Insulin resistance:** One hormone that aids in controlling blood sugar levels is insulin. Consuming large amounts of sugar regularly can cause insulin resistance, which raises the risk of heart disease. Because added sugar is metabolized differently by the body than sugar in entire foods, it is more damaging. High-added sugar diets cause our

blood sugar levels to rise sharply. The body converts and stores extra sugar as fat if it cannot use it as fuel, which furthers the cause of obesity.

3.   **Diabetes type 2:** Type 2 diabetes can eventually result from insulin resistance, which drives the pancreas to generate more insulin. Diabetes increases the risk of heart disease, stroke, and other cardiovascular diseases in people.

4.   **Gaining weight:** Soft drinks and packaged snacks are two examples of meals and beverages with a lot of added sugar that are high in calories but low in nutritious content. These "empty calories" mount up fast and play a part in excess weight gain, raising the risk of diseases like high blood pressure and cholesterol.

5.   **High blood pressure:** Diets heavy in sugar have been linked to elevated blood pressure, which is a major risk factor for stroke and heart disease.

Chapter 2

Benefits of zero sugar diet for 30 days

A common belief is that sugar is bad for our health. Ultimately, consuming excessive amounts of sugary snacks can lead to dental damage and weight gain. Eating too much sugar has been linked to obesity, diabetes, cardiovascular disease, and metabolic problems, according to a February 2023 study that was published in the National Library of Medicine. Hence, it makes sense to store cookies, pastries, brownies, cakes, ice cream, doughnuts, and toffee in storage. However, there exist alternative methods for ingesting sugar. You regularly consume tea along with other beverages. What if you avoided sweets for thirty days?

Eliminating sugar, or any other food category, from your diet is not a healthy option. Portion control and avoiding excess of any one food are the best ways to attain a balanced diet. According to Singhal, sugar offers calories but is devoid of important elements.

Among other things, consuming sugary food might cause you to overeat and deplete your diet of vital vitamins and minerals. The following are some advantages of giving up sugar for a month:

> **Better mental and emotional health**

Mental clarity and mood swings can both be positively impacted by stable blood sugar levels. Another benefit of cutting off sugar is improved psychological wellness. This is because consuming more added sugar is linked to a markedly increased risk of having episodes of anxiety, depression, and other mental health problems. The higher glycemic index of sugar is thought to be the cause of this inflammation in the brain, but it's crucial to note that studies indicate that consumption of added sugars—rather than natural sugars or total carbohydrates—appears to be the main culprit.

Reducing your sugar intake might also aid in maintaining memory function as you age. Researchers discovered a correlation between high sugar intake and the occurrence and severity of memory impairment in a 2020 cross-sectional study including 3,623 Americans 60 years of age and older that was published in the journal Nutrients. (Diets heavy in carbohydrates and total fat have also been linked similarly.) According to some research, memory issues in the hippocampus may be caused by increased inflammation in the brain. Sugar has also been connected to cardiovascular illness and type 2 diabetes; two diseases that have been associated with cognitive decline.

> **Healthier gut**

Cutting back on sugar can help support a healthier gut environment because consuming too much sugar can upset the balance of gut flora

> **Increased vitality**

When there are no blood sugar highs and lows, energy levels usually stabilize over the course of the day. Nearly all major lifestyle and age-related diseases, such as arthritis, GI problems, and metabolic syndrome, have been related to chronic, low-grade inflammation. High sugar consumption alters the balance of intestinal bacteria in mice, boosting the kind with pro-inflammatory characteristics, according to studies. A 2018 systematic review of 13 research including over 1,100 individuals revealed that all forms of added sugars (fructose, sucrose, glucose, and HFCS) increased levels of C-reactive protein, a crucial indicator of inflammation, despite the paucity and ongoing evolution of the data in human studies. A major dietary component known to increase chronic inflammation is added sugars. Chronic inflammation is an undesirable and aberrant immunological response in the body that results in an overactive immune system. Excessive use of added sugars has been shown to exacerbate inflammation, according to a review published in Frontiers in Immunology in 2022. Eliminating additional sugars can both reduce and prevent inflammation that already exists. This enhances immune system performance overall, enabling the body to combat infections more successfully and lessening the likelihood of disease.

> **Improved blood sugar levels**

A 30-day sugar fast can help normalize blood sugar levels and lower the risk of type 2 diabetes and insulin resistance. Research has indicated that consuming large amounts of sugar, particularly in sweetened beverages, may raise the risk of Type 2 diabetes. Scientists attribute this, in large part, to the weight gain associated with high-calorie intake of added sugar. Obesity and excess weight are frequently associated with impaired insulin sensitivity and issues controlling blood sugar, which can result in Type 2 diabetes.

Reducing added sugars lowers your risk of diabetes by making it easier to control your weight and maintain blood glucose levels within safe ranges. This results from the fact that additional sugars contribute to a vicious cycle of events that alter hormones and metabolism and raise the risk of diabetes. additional sugars provide extra calories; eating too many calories causes weight gain; weight increase raises blood glucose levels from additional sugar consumption, which causes insulin resistance, which causes even more weight gain.

Conversely, though, is also true. Researchers discovered that individuals who substituted one daily sugary beverage or fruit juice with water or another type of unsweetened drink had a 10% lower chance of developing Type 2 diabetes later in life. This finding was made after pooling the data from three large prospective observational studies involving nearly 200,000 American men and women and published in Diabetes Care in 2019. Therefore, breaking this loop and lowering your risk mostly depends on reducing additional sugars.

➢ **Weight loss**

Cutting less on sugar or abstaining from it for a month can help you lose weight since it gets rid of empty calories and makes overeating less likely. Consuming the same foods without the extra sugars that are typically present lowers your overall calorie consumption, which may make it simpler to lose weight and keep it off. Overindulgence in added sugars is linked to overweight and obesity, according to an analysis of the data from a 2021 Clinical Diabetes research. The impact of additional sugars on body weight is probably not particularly noteworthy. The only factor that matters is too many calories, while simple carbohydrates' lower satiation level might also be important. You can save hundreds of calories without consuming less food by replacing high-sugar items with low- or no-sugar options. Examples of these items include yogurt, breakfast cereal, and beverages.

> **Improved oral health**

Reducing sugar intake can help you avoid cavities and gum disease while also improving your oral health. Since you were a child, you have been told that sugar leads to tooth decay. If left unbrushed or unwashed, the sugar and other carbohydrates on your teeth feed oral bacteria, which then produces an acid that erodes the enamel's mineral content and finally causes a hole. Caries are linked to added sugars, not naturally occurring sugar-containing foods like apples.

➢ Reduced risk of chronic diseases

According to the experts, cutting back on sugar may reduce the chance of acquiring chronic illnesses like heart disease.

➢ Clearer skin

Because consuming large amounts of sugar has been connected to acne and other skin problems, some people may see improvements in the health of their skin. Reducing added sugar consumption and maintaining appropriate blood glucose levels may help to delay the aging process of the skin. An elevated sugar intake triggers the generation of AGEs, or advanced glycation end products, which are linked to a sped-up aging process of the skin. Research indicates that reducing sugar consumption may considerably slow down the aging effects of AGEs on the skin, particularly if your diet is high in fruits and vegetables.

> **Sugar Detox Will Reduce Your Cravings**

Regular consumption of sugar-filled foods and drinks increases cravings. This is because sugar activates the brain's reward center by releasing dopamine, which has a similar effect to that of addictive medications. This is why cutting out sugar for a few days can often result in moderate withdrawal symptoms including headaches, anxiety, and stronger-than-normal sugar cravings. After a few days, though, cravings for sweet, high-carb foods should start to decline dramatically.

Rather than stopping sugar completely, think about reducing your intake gradually to reduce any negative consequences.

➤ Your Energy Level Will Increase

One of the more noticeable benefits you might experience right away is a general improvement in energy, which is mostly brought on by fewer blood sugar highs and lows. While sugar may provide a brief spike in energy, it also causes a significant drop in blood sugar levels, which leaves you feeling drained, irritable, and a little hungrier. Longer-lasting, more consistent energy comes from swapping those added sugar calories for complex carbohydrates and foods like fruit that naturally include sugar and fiber. Your longer, more peaceful sleep—a benefit associated with consuming fewer added sugars—may also be contributing to your increased energy.

➤ Your Appetite and Hunger Will Decrease

An important hormone in controlling appetite is leptin. It provides the brain with guidance on when to eat, when to stop eating, and how fast or slow to speed up metabolism. However, the body becomes less sensitive to the signal that you are full when you develop insulin resistance and fat. Eliminating added sugars is a crucial step in enhancing glucose regulation, which gradually increases leptin activity in the body.

Chapter 3

What is the acceptable amount of sugar?

What is the appropriate amount of added sugar if 24 tablespoons a day is too much? Since sugar is not a necessary food in your diet, it's difficult to say. A formal sugar recommendation has not been released by the Institute of Medicine, which establishes Recommended Dietary Allowances, or RDAs.

Nonetheless, the American Heart Association advises men and women to limit their daily intake of added sugar to 150 calories (or roughly 9 teaspoons or 36 grams) for males and 100 calories (or approximately 6 teaspoons or 24 grams) for women. That is approximately equivalent to one 12-ounce can of Coke.

Taking out added sugar

Among the greatest methods to keep an eye on how much-added sugar you eat is to read food labels. When you come across any of the following names for added sugar, try to steer clear of them or reduce the quantity or frequency of the meals that contain them:

- ❖ syrup sugar molecules ending in "ose" (dextrose, fructose, glucose, lactose, maltose, sucrose).
- ❖ Molasses
- ❖ Malt sugar
- ❖ Invert sugar
- ❖ High-fructose corn syrup
- ❖ Honey
- ❖ Brown sugar
- ❖ Corn sweetener
- ❖ Corn syrup
- ❖ Fruit juice concentrates

Grams are frequently used to indicate total sugar, which includes added sugar. Take note of the overall number of servings as well as the grams of sugar in each serving. Even though it only lists 5 grams of sugar per serving, if three or four servings are typical, you might easily consume 20 grams of sugar, which is a significant quantity of added sugar.

Additionally, monitor how much sugar you include in your meals and drinks. Coffee and tea are among the liquids that contribute around half of the added sugar. Approximately two-thirds of coffee drinkers and one-third of tea drinkers added sugar or sweet flavorings to their beverages, according to a May 2017 Public Health research. The researchers also discovered that added sugar accounted for more than 60% of the calories in their drinks.

How can governments lower the amount of sugar that people eat or consume?

❖ Enhance accredited nutrition and health education for those who have the power to affect the dietary preferences of the general public.

❖ Continually educate people about health.

- ❖ Limit the advertising of goods that have added sugar, particularly beverages.
- ❖ Establish guidelines for all food and beverages provided by institutions supported by the government.
- ❖ Rethink sugary meals and beverages to reduce consumption.
- ❖ Limit the promotion, sponsorship, and advertising of any food and beverages that include added sugar in all media channels.

Which foods are beneficial for regulating and lowering blood sugar?

Low-GI foods may assist individuals in controlling or lowering their blood sugar levels. Nuts, legumes, whole grains, some fruits, non-starchy veggies, and lean proteins are a few examples.

Foods and drinks that the body absorbs slowly are frequently better for diabetics since they prevent blood sugar rises and falls. These foods may be referred to as low-GI by medical practitioners. The GI calculates how different foods affect blood sugar levels.

Foods having a low to medium GI score may be of interest to those who are trying to control their blood sugar levels. For a balanced diet, people can also combine meals with different GI scores, such as low and high.

In an emergency involving diabetes, there is no proof, nevertheless, that consuming a particular kind of food will lower blood sugar levels.

The top foods for those trying to keep their blood sugar levels in check are listed below.

Breads to eat

- ✓ whole wheat, particularly that which has been stone-ground
- ✓ Pumpernickel
- ✓ Bread baked using ancient grains like einkorn and emmer

✓ Rye

✓ Bread manufactured with fewer processed grains

Breads to avoid when maintaining zero sugar for 30 days

✓ Raisin toast with fruit bread

✓ Sugar-infused bread

✓ Bagels

✓ White bread

✓ Breads produced using finely ground or refined grains

Most nuts and seeds

Nuts have a low GI and are incredibly high in dietary fiber.

Nuts are also a good source of unsaturated fatty acids, plant protein, and other nutrients such as:

✓ Minerals, like potassium and magnesium

✓ Vitamins with antioxidants

✓ Plant-based compounds, such as flavonoids

Chapter 4

Foods to eat and foods to avoid when maintaining zero sugar for 30 days

While most 30-day no-sugar challenges prohibit similar items, the particular guidelines you follow may differ depending on the program you choose to adhere to.

Foods you should stay away from

People are advised to limit foods and beverages high in added sugars during a 30-day no-sugar challenge, such as:

- **Sugary breakfast foods:** bars, granola, cereals with added sugar, and flavored oatmeal

- **Candy:** caramels, gummy candy, and chocolate

- **Sugary alcoholic beverages:** mixed drinks, alcoholic beverages in cans with added sweetness, and liquor

- **Sugary baked goods:** sugar-filled cakes, doughnuts, cookies, and bread

- **Sweeteners:** table sugar, honey, coconut sugar, agave, maple syrup, and corn syrup

Ketchup, honey mustard, barbecue sauce, and coffee creamer Ketchup, honey mustard, barbecue sauce, and coffee creamer

Furthermore, the majority of no-sugar challenges advise against using low- or no-calorie artificial and organically derived sweeteners like Equal, Splenda, stevia, and monk fruit.

It's generally advised to avoid refined grains as much as possible and switch to whole-grain goods that don't include added sugars, such as white rice, pasta, and bread.

Food items to consume

Participants in the zero-sugar for a 30-day challenge are urged to eat a variety of complete, nutrient-dense foods, such as:

- **Unsweetened beverages:** Tea, water, sparkling water, and coffee without sugar
- **Vegetables:** Broccoli, cauliflower, spinach, sweet potatoes, carrots, asparagus, and zucchini, among others.
- **Frits:** fruits such as grapefruit, oranges, berries, grapes, and cherries.
- **Proteins:** eggs, meat, tofu, chicken, fish, etc.
- **Healthy fat sources:** avocados, egg yolks, almonds, seeds, olive oil, plain yogurt, etc.
- **Complex carb sources:** brown rice, quinoa, butternut squash, sweet potatoes, and so forth.

Are there drawbacks?

As long as you reduce added sugar consumption sensibly and combine it with a nutritious diet throughout the 30-day challenge, there are no negative physical health repercussions to be concerned about.

Like any restrictive food plan, no added sugar challenges could, however, cause some people to develop bad eating habits.

For instance, after taking part in this kind of challenge, some people could discover that they have established dangerous eating rules around items they used to enjoy or an obsessive obsession with healthy food.

Furthermore, it is troublesome to prioritize short-term restriction when long-term, permanent dietary and lifestyle changes are more crucial for overall health.

Reverting to a high-sugar diet after 30 days of no added sugar can negate the health advantages of cutting back on added sugar.

Chapter 5

Techniques that are sustainable for reducing sugar intake

If you're going to do a 30-day no-sugar challenge, utilize that time to figure out what meals and drinks make up the majority of your added sugar intake.

This will assist you in reducing your usage of those sources when the 30-day challenge is over.

While most people find it impractical, try not to focus on giving up all sources of added sugar permanently after the challenge. Rather, try making the shift to a long-term, health-conscious diet that is high in wholesome foods and low in added sugars.

Remember that you can design your challenge to emphasize cutting back on added sugar, rather than eliminating it. For those who now consume a large amount of added sugar, this might be a better option.

Try cutting back on your soda consumption by one can per week for a month, for instance, if you presently drink four cans a day. This can assist you in realistically reducing your intake of added sugar gradually.

Finally, it's critical to realize that your long-term health should always come first.

Try adopting a diet that feeds your body and permits you to occasionally indulge in your favorite foods, rather than focusing on eliminating particular meals or drinks.

This has far more of an impact on general health than any 30-day challenge could ever have.

Tips to remove sugar from meals for 30 days

Mango, pineapple, strawberry, and other fruits are high in sugar content. You don't have to exclude fruits from your no-sugar diet entirely. Fruits are naturally sweet, but they also provide important vitamins, minerals, fiber, and antioxidants that are good for you.

In general, modest fruit eating is advised, according to health experts. According to the expert, all of the natural sugars included in whole fruits are aided in slowing down the bloodstream's absorption of sugar by their fiber content. This lessens the effect on blood sugar levels. Fruits include elements that are very beneficial to health. They support healthy digestion, the immune system, and the heart.

However, keep an eye on portion sizes and steer clear of consuming excessive amounts of dried fruits and fruit liquids. These sugar sources are concentrated and lack the fiber that comes from entire fruits.

Here's how to reduce sugar intake:

- **Select whole foods**

Expert advises emphasizing complete, unprocessed foods including fruits, vegetables, whole grains, lean meats, and healthy fats.

No processing or refining has been done to whole foods. Additionally, they don't include any artificial ingredients or additions. Whole fruits, legumes, whole grains, veggies, and bone-in meat are some examples of these foods.

Extremely processed foods are at the other extreme of the range. It is difficult to restrict your intake of these prepared foods because they are made with mixtures of salt, sugar, fat, and additives that are meant to taste great.

Foods like chips, sugary cereals, soft drinks, and fast meals are examples of ultra-processed foods.

The average American's diet contains almost 90% of added sugars from ultra-processed foods and only 8.7% from home-cooked meals made with real foods.

When at all feasible, try cooking from scratch to stay away from added sugars. You are not required to prepare complex meals. You can achieve great outcomes with easy preparations like marinated meats and roasted vegetables.

- **Steer clear of beverages with added sugar**

Give up sugary beverages including soda, fruit juices, and coffee or tea that has been sweetened. Choose water, herbal tea, or just plain coffee in its place.

There are cereals for breakfast that include a lot of added sugar. According to one assessment, more than half the weight of some of the most well-liked ones had extra sugar.

A cereal in the study had 88% sugar by weight, with each serving containing more than 12 teaspoons (50 grams).

Furthermore, granola—which is typically touted as a nutritious food—was discovered to have an average of more sugar than any other cereal.

Breakfast staples like waffles, pancakes, muffins, and jams are also laden with added sugar.

Try these low-sugar breakfast ideas instead of saving those sugary ones for special occasions:

✓ avocado on whole-grain toast

✓ Oatmeal with fresh fruit added for sweetness

✓ Scrambled eggs with cheese and vegetables

✓ Greek yogurt paired with almonds and fruit

- **Read labels**

Look at the food labels and steer clear of anything that has "added sugars." Pay attention to components such as corn syrup, high fructose corn syrup, sucrose, and other sugar derivatives.

It takes more than just avoiding sweet meals to reduce your sugar intake. It can conceal itself in strange meals like oats and ketchup, as you have already seen.

Thankfully, food makers must now list additional sugars on product labels. Foods that include added sugars will have a list of total carbohydrates under that category.

Another option is to look for sugar in the ingredient list. Ingredients are listed from the largest amount to the lowest amount utilized by weight, so the more sugar that shows higher on the ingredient list, the more sugar the item contains.

On food labels, added sugar is referred to by more than 50 terms, making it harder to identify. These are a few of the most typical ones:

- ✓ dextrose
- ✓ invert sugar
- ✓ high fructose corn syrup
- ✓ cane sugar or cane juice
- ✓ rice syrup
- ✓ caramel
- ✓ molasses
- ✓ maltose

- **Choose your snacks carefully**

Select nutritious snacks over sugary ones, such as nuts, seeds, yogurt, or fresh fruit.

Just watch out for hidden sugar sources in the foods you eat, especially when dining out or consuming packaged goods. Foods that are processed sometimes have a "health halo." They appear healthy at first appearance, and their marketing may utilize terms like "natural" or "wholesome" to make them appear healthier than they are.

It may surprise you to learn that some snacks, such as protein bars, granola bars, and dried fruit, can have as much sugar as candy and chocolate bars.

One such example is dried fruit. It's loaded with antioxidants, minerals, and fiber. To avoid overindulging, you should moderate your intake as it also includes high amounts of natural sugar (and certain types may be "candied" with additional added sugar).

Here are some options for sugar-free, healthful snacks:

- ✓ fresh fruit
- ✓ No added sugar jerky
- ✓ seeds and nuts
- ✓ hard-boiled eggs

- **Prepare meals at home**

Cooking at home allows you to be in charge of the ingredients and keeps hidden sweets at bay.

- **Use natural sweeteners with no calories instead**

Sucralose and aspartame are only two examples of the sugar- and calorie-free artificial sweeteners available on the market.

On the other hand, these artificial sweeteners may be connected to dysbiosis in the gut flora, which can result in impaired regulation of blood sugar, heightened appetite, and weight gain. Because of this, it might be best to stay away from artificial sweeteners as well.

Some alternative natural sweeteners without calories seem promising. Stevia, erythritol, monk fruit, and allulose are a few of these.

Though some processing occurs before they reach your neighborhood grocery shop, they are entirely naturally derived. Research on these sugar substitutes is still ongoing.

- **Keep high-sugar goods out of the house as much as possible**

You could be more inclined to eat high-sugar items if you have them around the house. If you only need to reach the cupboard or refrigerator to obtain a sugar fix, it will require a lot of self-control to stop yourself.

Have a strategy in place for when sugar cravings occur, though, as it can be challenging to keep some items out of the house if you live with others. Research has demonstrated the powerful effects of diversions, like solving puzzles, in lowering cravings.

If it doesn't work, consider keeping some low-sugar, healthful snacks on hand to munch on.

- **Get enough sleep**

Your health must have healthy sleeping habits. Inadequate sleep has been connected to obesity, impaired immune system function, depression, and poor focus.

On the other hand, sleep deprivation may also influence your dietary choices, making you more likely to eat foods heavy in calories, fat, sugar, and salt.

In one study, those who stayed up late and didn't get enough sleep consumed more calories, soda, fast food, and fruits and vegetables than those who went to bed earlier and slept through the entire night.

Additionally, a recent observational study found that postmenopausal women who had larger intakes of added sugar had a higher risk of sleeplessness.

Getting more sleep could give you more control over your eating habits if you're finding it difficult to avoid choosing foods high in sugar.

Conclusion

An excessive amount of added sugar in the diet has been linked to several chronic illnesses, including obesity, type 2 diabetes, cancer, and heart disease.

Limiting sugar intake from obvious sources (such as desserts and drinks) is vital, but you should also be mindful of sugar hiding in some other typical meals (such as sauces, low-fat foods, and processed snacks).

Make the switch to a whole-foods-based diet from highly processed ones if you want complete control over how much-added sugar you consume.

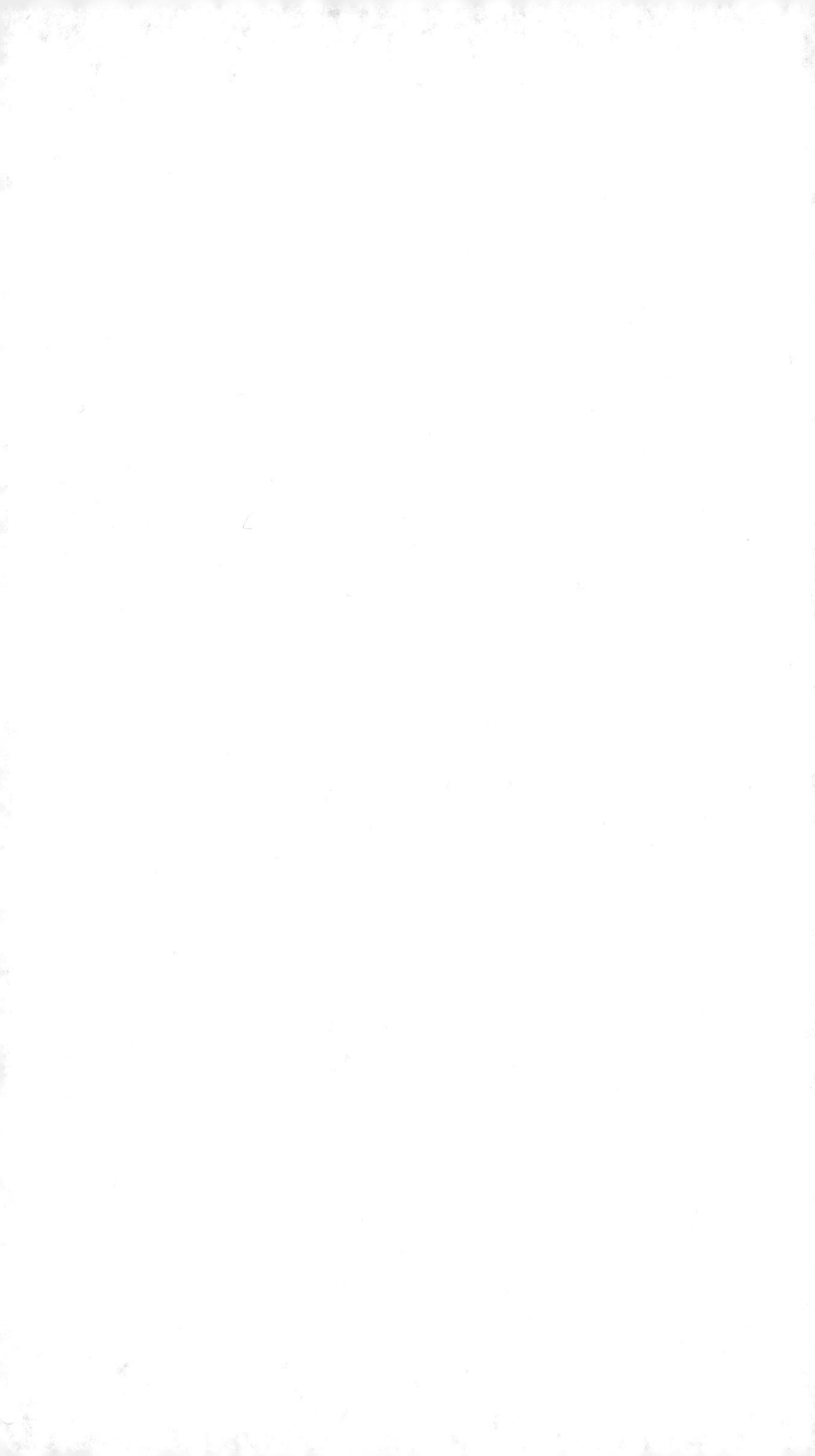

www.ingramcontent.com/pod-product-compliance
Lightning Source LLC
Chambersburg PA
CBHW070736260726
48660CB00007B/2876